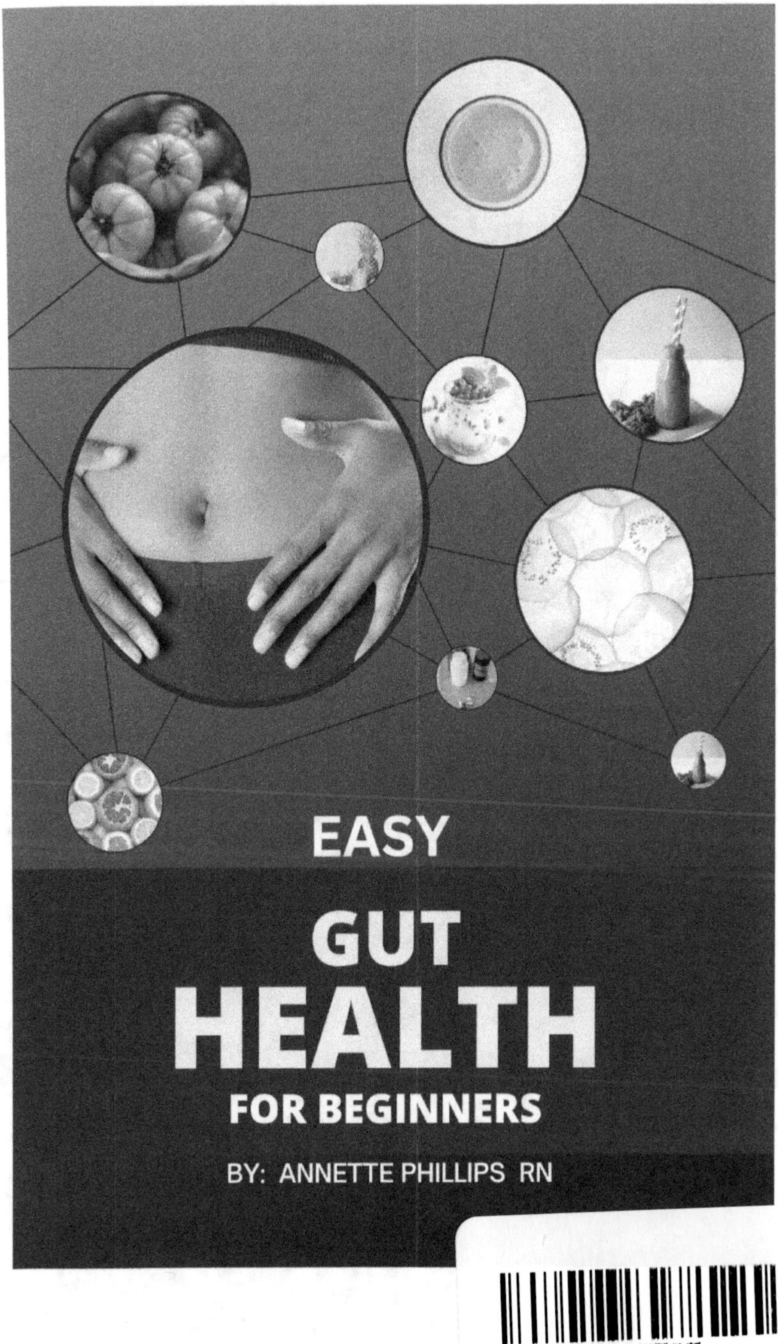

EASY

GUT
HEALTH

FOR BEGINNERS

BY: ANNETTE PHILLIPS RN

Annette Phillips

Easy GUT HEALTH

a beginner's guide

Copyright © 2023 by Annette Phillips

All rights reserved. No part of this publication may be reproduced, stored or transmitted in any form or by any means, electronic, mechanical, photocopying, recording, scanning, or otherwise without written permission from the publisher. It is illegal to copy this book, post it to a website, or distribute it by any other means without permission.

Annette Phillips asserts the moral right to be identified as the author of this work.

Annette Phillips has no responsibility for the persistence or accuracy of URLs for external or third-party Internet Websites referred to in this publication and does not guarantee that any content on such Websites is, or will remain, accurate or appropriate.

Designations used by companies to distinguish their products are often claimed as trademarks. All brand names and product names used in this book and on its cover are trade names, service marks, trademarks and registered trademarks of their respective owners. The publishers and the book are not associated with any product or vendor mentioned in this book. None of the companies referenced within the book have endorsed the book.

First edition

This book was professionally typeset on Reedsy

Find out more at reedsy.com

Contents

    1.

    2.

    3.

    4.

    5.

    6.

    7.

    8.

1

Introduction

Gut health, although often overlooked or ignored, plays a crucial role in our overall well-being. The state of the gut affects not only our digestion but also our immune system, mental health, and even skin conditions. Understanding the importance of gut health and learning how to improve it can have far-reaching benefits for our complete health.

This book will explore the intricate workings of the digestive system. It will also uncover the role of the gut microbiome, the community of bacteria and other microorganisms that reside within the intestines and directly impact all of our organs. There are various factors that can influence gut health, such as diet, lifestyle choices, medications, and stress, to name a few.

Recognizing the signs and symptoms of poor gut health, ranging from digestive issues to food intolerance and immune system problems is of primary importance. Effective strategies for improving gut health are included.

Healing the gut is possible and surprisingly simple. This book is a quick, condensed guide to gut health. Also, common questions and misconceptions about gut health will be explored. Evidence-based information will guide you on your path to health.

By the end of this book, you will have an understanding of the importance of gut health and a toolkit of strategies to support and improve it. I encourage you to prioritize your gut health and start on a transformative journey toward a healthier you.

2

The Digestive System

Navigating the Intricate Terrain of Your Gut: The Magnificent Digestive System.

Let's start by marveling at the wonder that is your digestive system. Picture it as a bustling metropolis, complete with intricate networks of highways and byways, all working together to ensure the smooth passage of nutrients and waste. From the moment food enters your mouth until it exits as waste, your digestive system is a well-orchestrated symphony of processes.

Now, let's meet the key players in this grand production. First, we have the mouth, where the adventure begins. Here, chewing and saliva and enzymes begin the process of breaking down food into smaller components. Next, the food travels down your esophagus and enters the stomach, a muscular pouch that churns and mixes the food with gastric juices. Next is the small intestine stretching out like a winding road. This remarkable organ is where the magic happens. It's here that nutrients from the broken-down food are absorbed into the bloodstream, providing fuel for your body's many functions. There are three sections of the small intestine—the duodenum, jejunum, and ileum. Each of these sections has a specific functions in the process of digestion and nutrient absorption:

The duodenum is the first and shortest section of the small intestine. Its primary function is to receive partially digested food from the stomach and mix it with digestive enzymes and bile from the liver and gallbladder. The duodenum plays a crucial role in breaking down food further, particularly proteins, carbohydrates, and fats. It also helps to neutralize the acidic stomach contents, allowing for optimal enzyme activity.

The jejunum is the middle section of the small intestine, located between the duodenum and the ileum. It is responsible for the majority of nutrient absorption. The inner lining of the jejunum contains finger-like projections called villi, which increase the surface area available for absorption. Nutrients, including carbohydrates, proteins, fats, vitamins, and minerals, are absorbed into the bloodstream through the cells lining the jejunum and transported to various organs and tissues for energy and other essential functions.

The ileum is the final and longest section of the small intestine, connecting to the large intestine (colon). While some nutrient absorption occurs in the ileum, its primary role is to absorb bile salts, vitamin B12, and any remaining nutrients that were not absorbed in the jejunum. The ileum also plays a role in the reabsorption of water and electrolytes before the remaining waste material moves into the large intestine for further processing.

Overall, the duodenum, ileum, and jejunum work together to break down food, extract nutrients, and facilitate their absorption into the bloodstream. This process is essential for providing the body with the energy and resources it needs to function properly. At the distal end is the intestine known as the colon. This is where water is absorbed, and the remaining waste material is formed into stool. Fascinating gut bacteria reside in the large intestine and play a crucial role in digestion and overall health. The appendix, a small, mysterious organ that has puzzled scientists for centuries, is located off of the colon.

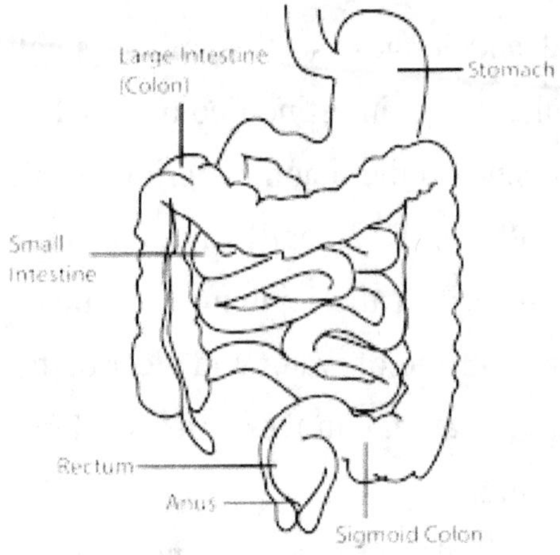

Finally, the digestive system concludes with the exit, or the rectum and anus, where waste material is stored and expelled from the body. Regular bowel movements are one of the signs of a healthy digestive system.

3

The Microbiome

Section 1:The Marvelous Microbiome:

1.

2. The gut microbiome refers to the vast community of microorganisms, including bacteria, viruses, fungi, and other microbes that reside in the gastrointestinal tract. Among these microbes, bacteria play a particularly significant role in maintaining gut health and function. Following are the functions of the biome

3. Digestion and nutrient absorption: bacteria in the gut microbiome aid in the breakdown and digestion of complex carbohydrates, fibers and other substances that the body cannot digest on its own. These bacteria produce enzymes that break down these compounds

into simpler forms, allowing the more effective absorption of these nutrients

4. Production of essential nutrients: certain bacteria in the gut biome have the ability to produce essential nutrients that our bodies require for optimal health. For example, vitamin K and certain B vitamins, which are crucial for various physiological processes.

5. Gut barrier function: The gut lining acts as a barrier between the contents of the gut and the rest of the body. Bacteria in the gut help maintain the integrity and function of this gut barrier by promoting the production of mucus and strengthening the tight junctions between gut cells. This barrier prevents harmful substances from entering the bloodstream, while allowing absorption of essential nutrients.

6. Immune system Regulation: Bacteria in the gut microbiome play a critical role in training and modulating our immune system. They interact with immune cells in the gut, helping to educate and fine-tune the immune response. This interaction is essential for maintaining a balanced immune system, preventing inappropriate immune reactions and protecting against pathogens.

7. Protection against pathogens: The presence of beneficial bacteria in the gut microbiome can help protect against harmful pathogens by competing with

them for resources. They also produce antimicrobial substances and stimulate the immune system to defend against potential invaders.

8. Regulation of metabolism and weight: Emerging research suggests that certain bacteria in the biome may play a role in regulating metabolism and body weight. Imbalances and decreased diversity of bacteria have been associated with conditions like obesity and metabolic disorders.

9. Brain-gut connection: The gut and the brain are connected through a bidirectional communication system known as the gut-brain axis. Bacteria in the biome produce various compounds and metabolites that can impact mood, cognition and behavior.

Section 2: Unveiling the Role of Gut Microorganisms

There is an enchanting world of the gut microbiome—a bustling community of microorganisms that inhabit your intestines. Prepare to be amazed by the vital role these tiny inhabitants play in shaping your overall health and well-being. Picture your gut as a thriving city, teeming with trillions of microscopic residents. Bacteria, viruses, fungi, and other microorganisms coexist in a delicate balance, forming a diverse and dynamic ecosystem. From aiding in digestion and nutrient absorption to synthesizing essential vitamins and minerals, these microorganisms in your gut are like industrious workers, tirelessly toiling away to keep your body running smoothly. It also shapes your immune system, influencing your mental health, and even affecting your weight and metabolism.

Section 3: The Dance of Balance: Maintaining a Healthy Microbiome

Just like any bustling city, the gut microbiome requires balance and harmony, proper diet and good lifestyle choices. The concept of dysbiosis, an imbalance in the gut microbial community causes a variety of maladies.

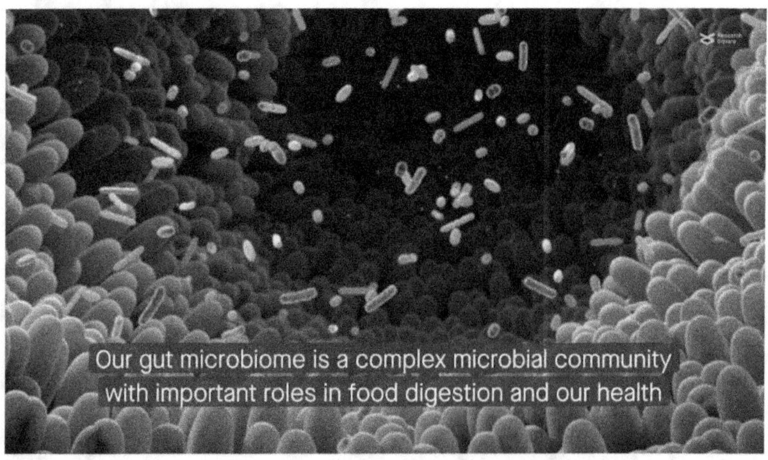

that serve as nourishment for beneficial gut bacteria are essential to consume. Additionally, probiotics, live microorganisms that can be consumed to promote a healthy gut microbiome should be consumed daily. Food sources rich in probiotics are yogurt, kefir, fermented foods and kimchi. There are also probiotics in pill form for convenience. It's important to purchase probiotics with live cell counts greater than 2 billion and varied strains represented such as lactobacillus rhamnosus and acidophilus.

To truly cultivate a thriving gut microbiome, we need to embrace a microbiome-friendly lifestyle by understanding the impact of stress, sleep, exercise, and environmental factors. By adopting healthy habits and making conscious choices, we can create an environment that fosters the growth of beneficial gut bacteria.

4

The Gut-Brain Axis

The Gut-Brain Connection: Unveiling the Intricate Pathway

Section 1: Enter the Gut-Brain Axis

Imagine a fiber optic communication superhighway stretching from your gut to your brain, buzzing with signals and messages. This is the gut-brain axis, a bidirectional communication pathway that involves the gut, the central nervous system, and the enteric (or gut) nervous system. The gut and brain are in constant dialogue.

Section 2: The Role of Neurotransmitters

Neurotransmitters, the chemical messengers of the brain, play a pivotal role in the gut-brain connection. The key neurotransmitters involved are serotonin, dopamine, and gamma-aminobutyric acid (GABA). These neurotransmitters are not only produced in the brain but also in the gut, influencing mood, cognition, and overall mental health.

Section 3: The Gut Microbiome's Influence

Beneficial gut bacteria produce neurotransmitters, including serotonin, which is often referred to as the "happy hormone." These neurotransmitters can cross the gut barrier, enter the bloodstream, and communicate with the brain, influencing our emotions and mental well-being. Moreover, the gut microbiome plays a vital role in regulating the immune system, which interacts closely with the brain. Imbalances in the gut microbiome can lead to chronic inflammation and immune dysregulation, which have been linked to mood disorders like depression and anxiety and also to countless auto-immune diseases.

Section 4: Stress and the Gut-Brain Connection

Stress, often referred to as the "silent killer," has a profound impact on the gut-brain connection. There is an intricate dance between stress and the gut. Chronic stress can disrupt the balance of gut bacteria, compromise the gut barrier, and impair gut function. This disruption can send signals to the brain, triggering a cascade of stress responses and potentially leading to mental health disorders.

Section 5: A Two-Way Street: Brain Influencing the Gut

Just as the gut influences the brain, the brain also has a significant impact on gut function. The central nervous system regulates gut motility, secretion, and blood flow. Stress, emotions, and mental state can all affect gut function, leading to symptoms like gastrointestinal distress and changes in appetite.

Section 6: Strategies for a Healthy Gut-Brain Connection

Some strategies for nurturing a healthy relationship between the gut and the brain are stress-management techniques, such as mindfulness meditation, deep breathing exercises, and engaging in activities that promote relaxation and well-being.

Diet also plays a crucial role in supporting a healthy gut-brain connection. Consuming a nutrient-dense diet, rich in whole foods and antioxidants, can provide the necessary building blocks for neurotransmitter production and support overall brain health. Additionally, incorporating gut-friendly foods, such as fermented foods and those rich in prebiotic fibers, can help nourish the gut microbiome and promote a healthy gut-brain axis.

Section 7: The Future of Gut-Brain Research

The study of the gut-brain connection is a rapidly evolving field, with potential implications and treatments for mental health, neurodegenerative diseases, and overall well-being. Ongoing research aims to uncover novel therapeutic approaches, including psychobiotics—probiotics specifically designed to influence the gut-brain axis—and targeted interventions that harness the power of the gut-brain connection. It is increasingly apparent that gut microbiome study could revolutionize healthcare treatments, making personalized medicine common-place and affordable.

5

Lifestyle Factors

Lifestyle

Section 1: Understanding the impact we can have on gut health.

It's imperative to note the importance of a diverse and balanced diet, rich in fiber, whole foods, and fermented foods. These dietary choices provide fuel for beneficial gut bacteria, promote regular bowel movements, and support a healthy gut microbiome.

Detrimental effects of a diet high in processed foods, added sugars, and unhealthy fats are the reality of today's Western society. Commercially prepared foods are most likely to have added ingredients to help their marketability. Such diets can disrupt the balance of gut bacteria, promote inflammation, and contribute to conditions like leaky gut syndrome and gastrointestinal disorders. It may be the best idea to prepare foods at home in order to increase awareness of what is consumed.

Section 2: The Role of Stress

Stress, a constant companion in our modern lives, has a profound impact on gut health. There is an intricate dance between stress and the gut. Chronic stress disrupts gut function, compromises the gut barrier, and alters the gut microbiome. These effects can contribute to conditions like irritable bowel syndrome (IBS) and gastrointestinal distress.

Stress-management techniques, such as mindfulness meditation, exercise, and engaging in activities that promote relaxation are very beneficial for the gut. These practices can help reduce stress levels and support a healthy gut environment.

Section 3: Medications and Gut Health

Certain medications can significantly impact gut health. Antibiotics, which can disrupt the balance of gut bacteria by killing both harmful and beneficial microbes should be avoided unless absolutely necessary for infections. Also the impact of non-steroidal anti-inflammatory drugs (NSAIDs) and proton pump inhibitors (PPIs) can contribute to gastrointestinal issues like dysbiosis and increased intestinal permeability (leaky gut).

While medications are sometimes necessary, there are strategies to mitigate their impact on gut health. This may include taking probiotics during and after antibiotic use, and exploring natural alternatives to manage conditions that may require long-term medication use.

Section 4: Environmental Factors and Gut Health

The environment we live in can greatly influence gut health. The impact of environmental toxins and pollutants, such as pesticides and heavy metals, are becoming more evident in modern society. These substances can disrupt the delicate balance of gut bacteria and contribute to inflammation and gut dysfunction.

As well as food, water quality has its impact on gut health. Consuming clean, filtered water can help reduce exposure to harmful contaminants and promote a healthy gut environment.

Section 5: Lifestyle Choices and Gut Health

Our lifestyle choices have a direct impact on gut health. Habits like smoking and excessive alcohol consumption can disrupt the gut microbiome, increase inflammation, and contribute to gastrointestinal disorders.

The benefits of regular physical activity has an impact on gut health, as exercise has been shown to support a diverse and healthy gut microbiome. The importance of getting adequate sleep cannot be overstated as sleep disturbances can negatively impact gut health and contribute to conditions like leaky gut syndrome.

Section 6: The Mind-Gut Connection

The gut-brain axis, a powerful bidirectional communication pathway, plays a significant role in gut health. Emotions, thoughts, and mental health can influence the gut and vice versa.

Emotions and stress have a profound impact on gut function. The gut is often referred to as our "second brain" because it contains a vast network of neurons, known as the enteric nervous system. This network communicates with the central nervous system, allowing emotions and stress to influence gut motility, secretion, and sensitivity.

Chronic stress and emotional disturbances can lead to gastrointestinal symptoms like stomach aches, bloating, and changes in bowel habits. Additionally, conditions like irritable bowel syndrome (IBS) have strong connections to stress and mental health disorders, highlighting the intricate relationship between the mind and the gut.

Studies have shown that individuals with mental health disorders often exhibit alterations in gut microbiota composition and increased intestinal permeability. Conversely, imbalances in gut bacteria and gut inflammation can also contribute to the development of mental health disorders.

Section 7: Diet

1. Incorporate Fiber-Rich Foods: Fiber acts as fuel for beneficial gut bacteria, promoting their growth and diversity. Emphasize whole grains, fruits, vegetables, legumes, and nuts in your diet to increase fiber intake.

2. Include Prebiotic Foods: Prebiotics are specific types of fiber that selectively nourish beneficial gut bacteria. Foods

like onions, garlic, leeks, asparagus, bananas, and Jerusalem artichokes are excellent sources of prebiotics.

3. Consume Fermented Foods: Fermented foods are rich in beneficial bacteria, known as probiotics. Include options like yogurt, kefir, sauerkraut, kimchi, and kombucha in your diet to introduce these live cultures.

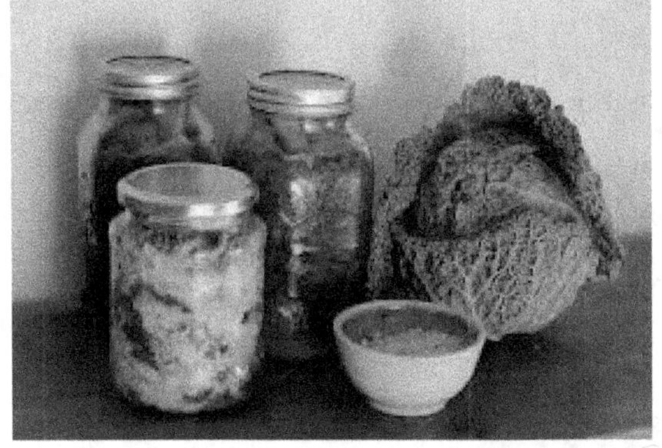

4. Limit Processed Foods: Processed foods are often low in fiber and high in added sugars, unhealthy fats, and artificial additives. Minimize their consumption as they can disrupt the balance of gut bacteria and contribute to gastrointestinal issues. These are generally the items in the middle aisles of the supermarket which are neatly packaged. The marketing on these items can be very enticing, but very few of these items are without sugar and other additives which are unhealthy for the gut . It may be most beneficial to shop only at the outer perimeter of the market for whole foods.

Section 8: Mind-Gut Connection and Mental Health

Understanding the mind-gut connection is crucial for improving gut health. Following are some strategies that focus on the interplay between mental health and gut health:

1. Cognitive-Behavioral Therapy (CBT): CBT is a therapeutic approach that helps individuals manage stress, anxiety, and depression. It can positively influence gut health by reducing stress levels and improving mental well-being.

2. Mindfulness-Based Techniques: Practices like meditation, deep breathing exercises, and yoga can help reduce stress and promote a healthier gut environment.

3. Seek Support: If you're experiencing symptoms related to gut health or mental health, seek support from healthcare professionals. They can provide guidance, therapies, and interventions tailored to your needs.

6

Signs and Symptoms

Signs and symptoms of poor gut health.

Section 1: Digestive Symptoms

Digestive symptoms are often the most apparent signs of poor gut health. These may include:

1. Bloating: Feeling excessively full or experiencing discomfort and distention in the abdomen.

2. Gas and Flatulence: Frequent passing of gas, often accompanied by a noticeable odor.

3. Abdominal Pain and Cramping: Unexplained pain or cramping in the abdominal region.

4. Diarrhea or Constipation: Frequent loose stools or difficulty passing stools

5. Heartburn and Acid Reflux: A burning sensation in the chest or throat, often after eating.

Section 2: Changes in Bowel Movement Habits

Observing changes in bowel movements can provide valuable insights into gut health. Look out for:

1. Irregular Bowel Movements: Inconsistent or unpredictable patterns of bowel movements.

2. Alternating Diarrhea and Constipation: Frequent shifts between loose stools and difficulty passing stools.

3. Persistent Diarrhea or Constipation: Experiencing prolonged episodes of diarrhea or constipation.

Section 3: Food Intolerances

Food intolerances can often be indicative of gut issues. Pay attention to:

1. Gluten Intolerance: Experiencing digestive discomfort, bloating, or bowel irregularities after consuming gluten-containing foods.

2. Lactose Intolerance: Experiencing digestive symptoms like bloating, gas, or diarrhea after consuming dairy products.

3. Other Food Sensitivities: Noticing adverse reactions or discomfort after consuming specific foods, such as nuts, eggs, or certain fruits and vegetables.

Section 4: Mood and Mental Health

The gut-brain connection can manifest in mood and mental health symptoms. Watch out for:

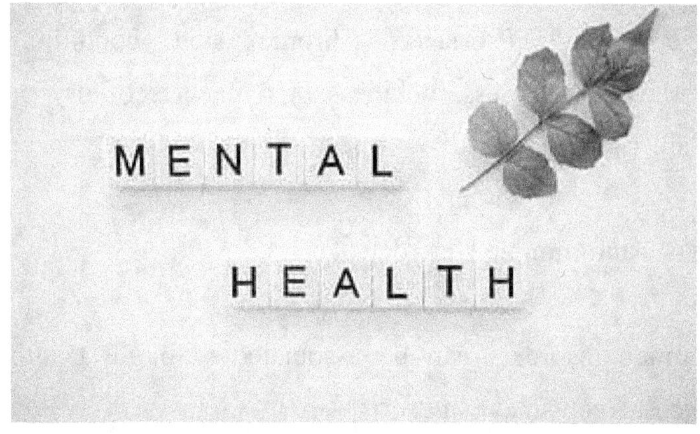

1. Anxiety and Depression: Experiencing prolonged feelings of anxiety, low mood, or persistent sadness.

2. Brain Fog: Difficulty concentrating, mental fatigue, or a feeling of clouded thinking.

3. Irritability and Mood Swings: Frequent changes in mood, ranging from irritability to sudden bursts of anger or sadness.

Section 5: Skin Conditions

Skin conditions can be linked to poor gut health. Look for:

1. Acne and Breakouts: Frequent or persistent acne, particularly on the face, back, or chest.

2. Eczema and Psoriasis: Chronic skin conditions characterized by redness, itchiness, and patches of dry or scaly skin.

Section 6: Autoimmune Disorders

Autoimmune disorders can be associated with gut health imbalances. Keep an eye out for:

1. Rheumatoid Arthritis: Joint pain, stiffness, and swelling due to inflammation.

2. Hashimoto's Thyroiditis: An autoimmune condition affecting the thyroid gland, often leading to hypothyroidism.

3. Inflammatory Bowel Disease (IBD): Chronic inflammation of the digestive tract, including conditions like Crohn's disease and ulcerative colitis.

It's essential to remember that these symptoms are not exclusive to poor gut health and can have various other causes. If you are experiencing any persistent or concerning symptoms, it is recommended to seek guidance from a healthcare professional for an accurate diagnosis and appropriate treatment.

By listening to the body's messages and recognizing these signs and symptoms, you can take proactive steps to improve gut health and overall well-being.

7

Supplements and Herbs

Gut Healing Supplements, Herbs, and Restoring Practices

There are various supplements, herbs, and practices that can aid in gut healing and restoration. These natural remedies can complement a healthy diet and lifestyle, supporting the balance of gut bacteria, reducing inflammation, and promoting overall gut health.

Section 1: Gut Healing Supplements

1. Probiotics: Probiotic supplements contain live bacteria strains that can help restore and maintain a healthy gut

microbiome. Look for a high-quality product with a variety of strains and a high colony-forming unit (CFU) count.

2. Digestive Enzymes: Digestive enzyme supplements can aid in the breakdown and absorption of nutrients, especially for those with digestive issues. Look for a broad-spectrum enzyme blend that includes protease, lipase , amylase and some include cellulase, bromelain and papain as well.

3. L-Glutamine: L-Glutamine is an amino acid that plays a crucial role in gut health and repair. It can help strengthen the gut lining, reduce inflammation, promote healing and support the growth of beneficial gut bacteria.

4. Slippery Elm: Slippery elm is an herb that has been traditionally used to soothe and heal the digestive tract. It forms a protective coating on that plays a crucial role in gut health and repair. It can help strengthen the gut lining, reduce inflammation, and support the growth of beneficial gut bacteria.

5. Marshmallow Root: Marshmallow root is another herb known for its soothing properties. It can help relieve inflammation in the gut, support the healing of the mucous membranes, and improve digestion.

Section 2: Gut Restoring Herbs and Practices

1. Aloe Vera: Aloe Vera gel has anti-inflammatory and healing properties that can benefit the gut. It can help reduce inflammation, soothe the digestive tract, and support gut healing.

2. Licorice Root: Licorice root is known for its anti-inflammatory properties and its ability to support gut health. It can help soothe the digestive tract, reduce inflammation, and promote a healthy gut lining.

3. Bone Broth: Bone broth is rich in nutrients and collagen, which can help heal and seal the gut lining. It also contains amino acids and minerals that support gut health and overall well-being. It can be made by simply boiling and seasoning the broth from any bones.

4. Intermittent Fasting: Intermittent fasting involves cycling between periods of eating and fasting. It can give the digestive system a break, reduce inflammation, and promote gut healing.

5. Mindful Eating: Practicing mindful eating involves paying attention to the process of eating, chewing food thoroughly,

and being present during meals. This can improve digestion, nutrient absorption, and overall gut health.

It's important to note that while these supplements, herbs, and practices can be beneficial for gut health, they may not be suitable for everyone. It's always recommended to consult with a healthcare professional or a qualified herbalist to determine the right approach for your specific needs and any potential interactions with medications or existing health conditions.

Remember that supplements and herbs should complement a healthy diet and lifestyle, rather than replace them. Prioritizing a balanced diet, stress management, regular exercise, and other lifestyle practices is crucial for long-term gut health and overall well-being.

8

Myths about Gut Health

Addressing Concerns and Misconceptions About Gut Health

Gut health is a topic that has gained significant attention in recent years, leading to various concerns and misconceptions. This chapter will address some common concerns and misconceptions surrounding gut health to provide clarity and accurate information.

Myth 1: All Digestive Issues Are Related to Gut Health

While the gut plays a crucial role in digestion, not all digestive issues are solely due to gut health. Other factors, such as food intolerance, medication side effects, hormonal imbalances, and stress, can also contribute to digestive problems. It's important to consider these factors and consult with a healthcare professional for an accurate diagnosis and appropriate treatment.

Myth 2: Probiotics Are the Only Solution for Gut Health

While probiotics can be beneficial for gut health, they are not the only solution. A holistic approach that includes a healthy diet, lifestyle modifications, stress management, and addressing underlying health conditions is essential. Probiotics are a tool in supporting a healthy gut microbiome, but they should be used in conjunction with other strategies for optimal gut health.

Myth 3: Gut Health Is Only About Digestion

Although the gut is primarily responsible for digestion, its impact extends beyond that. The gut-brain connection highlights the influence of gut health on mental health, mood regulation, and immune function. Poor gut health has been associated with conditions like depression, anxiety, and autoimmune disorders. Therefore, maintaining a healthy gut is crucial for overall well-being.

Myth 4: Gut Health Is Difficult to Improve

Improving gut health is not an insurmountable challenge. With the right knowledge and implementation of gut-friendly practices, it is possible to make positive changes. Focus on a balanced diet rich in fiber and fermented foods, manage stress levels, get regular exercise, and consider targeted supplements or herbs. Small, consistent steps can lead to significant improvements in gut health over time.

Myth 5: Gut Health Is the Same for Everyone

Each person's gut microbiome is unique, influenced by genetics, diet, lifestyle, and environmental factors. What works for one person may not work for another. It's crucial to listen to your body, experiment with different strategies, and pay attention to how specific foods or practices affect your gut health. Consulting with a healthcare professional or registered dietitian can provide personalized guidance based on your individual needs.

Myth 6: Gut Health Is Only Relevant for Digestive Issues

While gut health is directly linked to digestive issues, it also impacts overall health and well-being. A healthy gut microbiome plays a vital role in immune function, nutrient absorption, hormone regulation, and inflammation control.

Prioritizing gut health can have far-reaching benefits beyond digestion.

35

9

Key Points

Key takeaways

Everyone's journey to optimal gut health is unique, and it may require some trial and error to find the strategies that work best for you. With patience, persistence, and guidance from healthcare professionals, you can take proactive steps to support your gut health and overall well-being.

1. Embrace a Gut-Friendly Diet: Incorporate fiber-rich foods, fermented foods, and prebiotic-rich foods into your diet to support the growth of beneficial gut bacteria.

2. Consider Probiotics: Probiotic supplements can help restore and maintain a healthy gut microbiome. Look for a product with diverse strains and a high CFU count.

3. Manage Stress: Chronic stress can negatively impact gut health. Engage in stress-reducing activities like meditation, deep breathing exercises, and yoga.

4. Get Regular Exercise: Regular physical activity supports a diverse and healthy gut microbiome. Aim for at least 150 minutes of moderate-intensity exercise per week.

5. Optimize Digestion: Chew your food thoroughly, stay hydrated, and consider digestive enzyme supplements if needed to support proper digestion and absorption of nutrients.

6. Prioritize Sleep: Aim for 7-9 hours of quality sleep per night to promote a healthy gut microbiome and overall well-being.

7. Limit Alcohol and Smoking: Excessive alcohol consumption and smoking can disrupt gut health. Drink alcohol in moderation or consider eliminating it altogether, and seek support to quit smoking.

8. Minimize Exposure to Toxins: Be mindful of exposure to environmental toxins such as pesticides and household chemicals. Choose organic produce, use natural cleaning products, and filter your water when possible.

9. Address Digestive Issues Holistically: Consider underlying factors like food intolerances, medication side effects, and hormonal imbalances that can contribute to digestive problems. Consult with a healthcare professional for an accurate diagnosis and appropriate treatment.

10. Personalize Your Approach: Everyone's gut is unique, so it may take time and experimentation to find the strategies that work best for you. Listen to your body, seek professional guidance when needed, and make adjustments as necessary.

By implementing these key takeaways, you can take proactive steps to improve your gut health, support a healthy gut microbiome, and enhance your overall well-being. Remember that consistency and patience are key, as gut health improvements may take time. With a holistic approach and a focus on self-care, you can cultivate a healthier gut and enjoy the benefits it brings to your life.

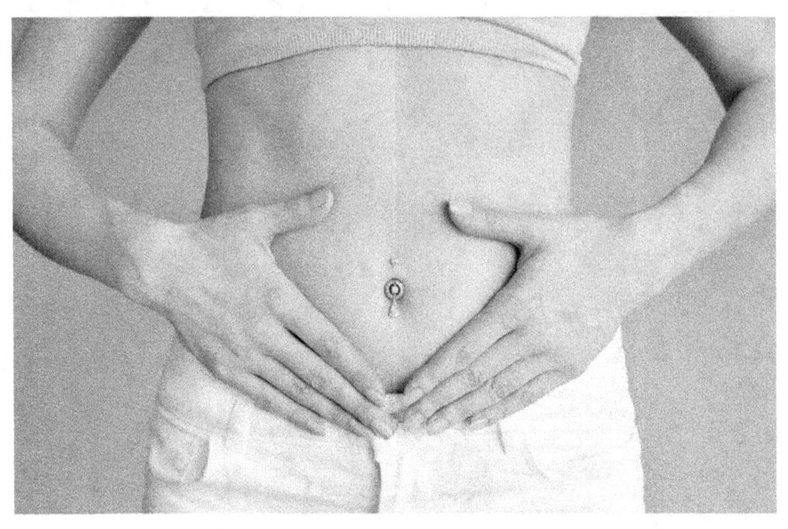